FEINGOLD DIET COOKBOOK

Over 100 Delicious Recipes to Support Your Feingold Diet Journey

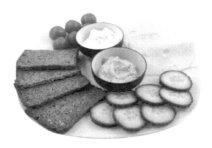

CHARLES MURRAY

Copyright
Copyright © 2023 by Charles Murray

All rights reserved. No part of this book may be
reproduced, stored in a retrieval system, or
transmitted in any form or by any means,
electronic, mechanical, photocopying,
recording, or otherwise, without the prior
written permission of the author.

This book is a work of non fiction. Names,
characters, places, and incidents are either the
product of the author's imagination or are used
fictitiously. Any resemblance to actual persons,
living or dead, or to actual events or locales is
entirely coincidental.

1

Table of content

INTRODUCTION

Tommy had a history of eating pickily. His parents made numerous attempts to get him to consume his vegetables, but he consistently refused to do so. Tommy's nutrition therefore mainly comprised of quick food, prepared foods, and sweet treats.

When Tommy's aunt paid him a call one day, she took note of his dietary patterns. She advised him to give the Feingold Diet a shot because it had helped her own children with ADHD. Tommy received a copy of the Feingold Diet Cookbook from her, and she suggested he attempt a few of the dishes.

Tommy was initially dubious, but he soon became fascinated by the vibrant images and detailed explanations of the recipes. He decided to give it a shot and began by baking some chicken fingers.

The chicken fingers were excellent, much to his delight! He was unable to comprehend how delicious and nutritious cuisine could be. He persisted in experimenting with more of the cookbook's recipes, making handmade pizza and spaghetti zucchini strands among them. He was loving testing out new cuisines, and each preparation was better than the one before it.

Tommy observed that he had more energy and felt better generally as he continued to consume more healthfully. He wasn't getting ill as frequently, and his concentration in the class had improved. He even began to look forward to shopping with his mother and selecting the fresh ingredients for his new go-to dishes.

Tommy's mother observed how much he had altered since he began eating better one day. When she questioned him about his motivation for the shift, he demonstrated the Feingold Diet Cookbook that his aunt had given him. The variety of recipes and the lovely photographs mesmerized her, and she decided to attempt some of the recipes for herself.

The entire family soon began consuming more healthfully and feeling better. They were experimenting with novel cuisines and having fun while preparing together. Tommy was thankful to the Feingold Diet Cookbook for setting him on this path because it had brought him serenity in knowing that he was caring for his body and his health.

Let's get back to the main introduction to this book.
Welcome to the Feingold Diet Cookbook, a thorough manual for wholesome and delectable dining that will transform the way you view food. The Feingold Diet is a cutting-edge regimen that emphasizes getting rid of unhealthy food chemicals and contaminants from your diet so

that you can consume healthful, nourishing foods that promote your general health and well-being.

This guidebook is your go-to source for delicious, simple-to-prepare dishes that are Feingold Diet-compatible. This guide has all the information you need to make delicious and wholesome meals that the whole family will enjoy, whether you're looking for morning suggestions, munchies, soups, salads, side dishes, main courses, sweets, or pastry recipes.

The Feingold Diet's guiding principles, including the kinds of food chemicals to avoid and the foods that are acceptable under the plan, will be covered in more detail in the parts that follow. We'll give you a list of cupboard essentials you'll need to prepare delectable Feingold Diet dishes as well as helpful advice on meal preparation and meal planning to make cooking simpler and more effective.

The cookbook's core section, with a broad variety of dishes for every situation and preference, will then be covered. This guide offers a plethora of choices to fit every taste and lifestyle, from quick and simple meals to substantial main dishes, from kid-friendly munchies to indulgent sweets.

This recipe is intended to encourage you to adopt the Feingold Diet and experience the benefits of a pure, nutritious diet. We are thrilled to share this recipe with you as a resource for reaching your health and well-being objectives because we firmly believe that a healthy diet is the cornerstone of good health. So let's get going and set out on our quest for a better, happier, and more mouthwatering existence!.

CHAPTER ONE: What is the Feingold Diet?

The Feingold Diet is an all-encompassing nutritional plan that emphasizes cutting out fake food chemicals and pesticides from the diet. The program, created by Dr. Benjamin Feingold in the 1970s, has grown in prominence as a means of enhancing general health and wellbeing, particularly in kids who might be susceptible to specific dietary chemicals.

The Feingold Diet is founded on the idea that some dietary chemicals, especially in children, can cause behavioral issues, cognitive challenges, and other health problems. The program concentrates on removing two types of additives: fake flavorings and manufactured food colors. These ingredients are frequently present in packed products like sweets, beverages, and many other prepared meals. The program also promotes the removal of some additives that are used to prolong the expiration life of many manufactured goods, such as BHA and BHT.

People who are sensitive to or hypersensitive to them, as well as those seeking to enhance their general health and wellbeing, are thought to profit from the removal of these chemicals. Children with ADHD or autism are frequently advised to follow the Feingold

Diet because it is thought that these children may be more susceptible to the negative effects of manufactured food ingredients.

The Feingold Diet places a strong emphasis on the intake of whole, natural foods in addition to the removal of dangerous food chemicals. The program advises people to avoid highly manufactured foods, which are frequently loaded with chemical substances and pesticides, and to make their own dinners from fresh. The diet plan places a strong emphasis on the intake of fresh produce, whole cereals, lean meats, and healthy lipids like avocado, almonds, and seeds.

The Feingold Diet stresses the value of removing dangerous food chemicals from the diet while boosting the intake of whole, natural foods. It is a comprehensive strategy to healthy nutrition. Individuals who adhere to this program may see improvements in their health, including better metabolism, better slumber, more vitality, and a decrease in the signs of conditions like ADHD or autism.

Importance of the Feingold Diet

We will thoroughly examine the Feingold Diet's numerous advantages in this part.

Improved Digestion:

The Feingold Diet can aid in improving digestion by removing fake chemicals and pesticides from the diet. Many of these chemicals have a history of contributing to gastrointestinal problems like swelling, flatulence, and diarrhea. People may experience improved gut health, such as better stool motions and fewer signs of irritable bowel syndrome, by eliminating these substances from their diet. (IBS).

Better slumber:

Many people who adhere to the Feingold Diet report having better slumber. This is due to the fact that some dietary ingredients, such as synthetic flavors and colors, can interfere with the body's normal slumber pattern. Eliminating these substances from the diet may improve sleep quality, allowing people to doze off more quickly and remain sleeping longer.

Boosted Energy:

The Feingold Diet places a strong emphasis on consuming whole, organic foods like fruits, veggies, whole cereals, and lean meats. These meals are nutrient-rich and can give the body the vitality it requires to operate at its best. People who adhere to the Feingold Diet may have more vitality, feel less fatigued, and perform better physically.

The Feingold Diet is frequently advised for kids with attention deficit hyperactivity disorder in order to lessen their symptoms. (ADHD). Many ADHD kids are susceptible to specific food chemicals, so removing them from the diet may help parents notice a decrease in their child's symptoms, like restlessness and recklessness.

Better Skin Health:

Some dietary chemicals, like synthetic stabilizers, have been related to skin conditions like dermatitis and pimples. People may experience better skin health, such as decreased redness and fewer acne, by removing these chemicals from their food.

Weight loss:

The Feingold Diet places a strong emphasis on eating whole, natural foods because they frequently have fewer calories and more minerals than manufactured foods. Individuals who adhere to this method may experience weight reduction or stabilization as well as a decreased chance of obesity and associated health problems.

Reduced Risk of Chronic Diseases:

The Feingold Diet places a strong emphasis on eating whole, natural foods because they are full of minerals and vitamins that can lower the risk of developing chronic illnesses like cancer, diabetes, and heart disease.

Better Mental Health:

Studies have shown a connection between certain dietary chemicals and mental illnesses like worry and melancholy. Individuals may experience better mental health, including decreased worry and enhanced happiness, by removing these substances from their food.

Increased Longevity:

Individuals who follow the Feingold Diet may see an improvement in their health, which may promote longer life expectancy and a higher standard of living in later years.

In general, those seeking to enhance their general health and wellbeing can profit greatly from the Feingold Diet. People may experience better digestion, better sleep, more energy, fewer ADHD symptoms, improved skin health, weight loss, lowered risk of chronic diseases, improved mental health, and increased longevity by cutting out artificial food additives and preservatives from their diet.

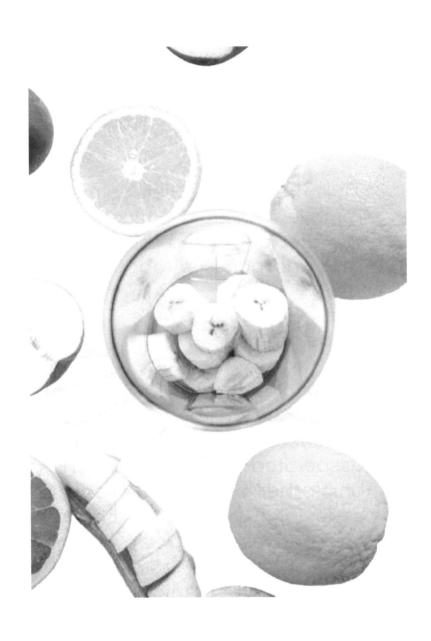

CHAPTER TWO: Feingold Diet Principles

The Feingold Diet aims to remove these chemicals from the diet and swap them out for real, unprocessed foods.

The Feingold Diet's guiding ideas are as follows:

Artificial food flavors are prohibited on the Feingold Diet because they have been associated with restlessness and other behavioral problems, especially in children. Alternatives include using natural culinary colorings like turmeric or beet juice.

Elimination of fake tastes: All artificial flavors are prohibited by the Feingold Diet because they may contain chemicals that have been related to harmful health effects. Instead, you can use natural flavorings like vanilla essence or lemon peel.

Preservatives are eliminated entirely on the Feingold Diet because they raise the risk of allergy responses, respiratory attacks, and other health problems. Instead, you can use natural stabilizers like vinegar or citric acid.

The Feingold Diet places a strong emphasis on the intake of whole, organic foods like fruits, veggies, whole cereals, and lean meats. These meals are nutrient-dense and give the body the minerals and energy it requires to operate at its best.

The Feingold Diet restricts the intake of manufactured foods, which are frequently loaded with chemical substances and pesticides. Instead, people are urged to cook their own dinners and treats with organic, whole foods.

Personalization: The Feingold Diet is aware that each person's body is unique and may respond to certain meals in a variety of ways. As a result, the software enables customization and urges users to monitor their responses to particular meals and modify their diet appropriately.

The Feingold Diet emphasizes the intake of whole, natural foods while removing fake chemicals and pesticides from the diet in order to encourage general health and wellbeing. By adhering to these rules, people may have better metabolism, better sleep, more energy, fewer ADHD signs, better physical health, weight reduction, lower chance of chronic illnesses, better mental health, and longer lifespans.

In a more detailed explanation, here are the diet principles:

Elimination of artificial colors:
The Feingold Diet emphasizes the removal of fake hues. Many manufactured foods contain artificial food flavors, which are

manmade compounds added to improve their look and allure to customers. These hues, which frequently come from coal ash or gasoline, have been connected to a number of harmful health impacts, especially in young people.

Artificial food colorings have been found in studies to make children's signs of ADHD and other behavioral problems worse. According to a research in The Lancet, ingesting fake food flavors and additives can make kids up to 30% more restless. Additional research has connected fake food coloring to a number of additional harmful health outcomes, such as allergens, asthma, and cancer.

Artificial food hues are prohibited by the Feingold Diet because it acknowledges their possible risks. Instead, the program places a strong emphasis on the use of natural dietary flavors that come from pure, unprocessed sources. For instance, turmeric can be used to give food a natural golden color, and beet juice can be used to give food a natural crimson color.

The health benefits of removing fake food hues from the diet are numerous. While people with allergens or asthma may experience a decrease in symptoms, children with ADHD may exhibit better conduct and concentration ability. Eliminating synthetic food dyes may also enhance general health and wellbeing by lowering exposure to dangerous substances and encouraging a diet rich in whole, natural foods.

The Feingold Diet's main tenet is the removal of fake hues because it can significantly improve health and wellbeing. People can improve their general health and lower their chance of adverse health impacts by opting to ingest natural food colors and avoiding manufactured foods that contain fake hues.

Elimination of artificial flavors:

One such ingredient that is banned from the diet according to the Feingold Diet's principals is artificial tastes.

Chemical substances known as artificial tastes are added to manufactured meals to improve their flavor and increase customer attraction. These tastes can contain a variety of chemical substances that have been related to harmful health impacts and are frequently taken from manufactured sources.

Research has shown that some fake tastes, especially those marketed to children, can trigger allergy responses and asthma. Some fake tastes have additionally been connected to other harmful health impacts, such as headaches, stomach difficulties, and behavioral issues.

Artificial tastes are not allowed on the Feingold Diet because of the possible risks they pose. Instead, the program places a strong emphasis on the use of natural flavorings that come from pure, unprocessed sources. For instance, orange peel can be used to add a natural citrus flavor to food, whereas vanilla essence can be used to contribute a natural vanilla flavor to food.

The health benefits of eliminating fake tastes from the food are numerous. Eliminating fake tastes can lessen symptoms and improve general health in people with allergies or asthma. Consuming natural tastes can also help people eat more whole, natural foods and ingest fewer toxic additives.

The Feingold Diet's main tenet is the removal of fake tastes because it can significantly improve health and wellbeing. People can improve their general health and lower their chance of adverse health effects by opting to consume natural flavorings and avoiding manufactured foods that contain fake flavors.

Elimination of preservatives:

Chemical substances called preservatives are added to manufactured goods to increase storage life and stop deterioration. While some additives have been related to harmful health impacts like allergy responses, stomach issues, and cancer, others may help keep food fresh and secure.

The Feingold Diet places a strong emphasis on the intake of whole, natural foods and the avoidance of chemical substances and preservatives, such as BHA, BHT, and TBHQ, which are popular food stabilizers. Instead, to preserve the freshness of goods, the program promotes the use of natural preservation techniques like preserving or chilling.

Eliminating additives from the food can improve health in a number of ways. In contrast to manufactured foods with additional additives, whole, natural foods are better for people's general health and wellbeing because they expose them to fewer toxic substances.

Additionally, removing additives can enhance the flavor and texture of food. Natural preservation techniques can help to keep the fresh and natural flavor of foods while preservatives can frequently give food a fake or manufactured flavor.

Overall, the Feingold Diet's key tenet of eliminating additives is crucial because it can significantly improve health and wellbeing. People can improve their general health and lower their chance of adverse health impacts by choosing to eat whole, natural foods and avoiding manufactured foods with additional additives.

Emphasis on whole, natural foods:

The Feingold Diet places a strong emphasis on eating whole, unprocessed foods to improve health and lower ingestion of dangerous chemicals and pesticides. This entails avoiding or drastically reducing the consumption of packed and processed foods in favor of naturally occurring, barely processed raw foods.

Whole, natural foods are those that have not undergone substantial processing or alteration and are in their original form. Fruits, veggies, whole cereals, lean meats, and healthful lipids are a few of these. People can take advantage of the minerals and fiber that whole, natural foods offer by selecting them, which can lower the chance of developing chronic illnesses like heart disease, diabetes, and obesity.

Additionally, eating whole, natural foods can aid in lowering the consumption of hazardous chemicals and substances that are frequently present in manufactured foods. The Feingold Diet, for instance, advises against chemical colors, tastes, and additives because they have been associated with adverse health impacts like allergens, asthma, and behavioral issues in children.

The Feingold Diet's focus on whole, natural meals is one of its guiding principles and can have a variety of beneficial impacts on health and wellbeing. People can improve their general health, lower their risk of developing chronic illnesses, and feel better bodily and psychologically by ingesting whole, natural foods rather than manufactured foods with additional chemicals and substances.

The Feingold Diet, in its entirety, stresses the value of consuming whole, natural foods as a way to enhance health and lessen consumption of hazardous chemicals and pesticides. Individuals can enhance their general health and well-being and lower their chance of adverse health impacts by switching to whole, natural meals.

Limited consumption of processed foods:

Limiting the intake of manufactured meals is one of the Feingold Diet's major tenets. Foods that have undergone changes from their natural form are referred to as processed foods. Usually, these changes are made to increase storage life or enhance taste or mouthfeel. Some people may have issues with the numerous substances and compounds that these meals frequently contain, such as fake colors, tastes, and preservatives.

The Feingold Diet seeks to lessen ingestion of these substances and chemicals, which may have a detrimental effect on some people's behavior and health, by restricting the consumption of manufactured foods. Instead, the diet promotes the intake of whole foods like fresh produce, whole cereals, lean meats, and veggies.

On the Feingold Diet, manufactured meals should generally be shunned as follows:

Sweets and salty nibbles
processed meats, such as picnic meats and hot dogs
Fast cuisine and ready meals
made products that have been packaged, like biscuits and snacks

dishes that are pre-packaged
and frozen

soda and other sweetened
beverages

It's crucial to remember that not
all manufactured meals are
inherently unhealthy. When
manufactured foods don't have
extra sweeteners or additives,
they can be healthful choices,
like packaged fruits and
veggies. The Feingold Diet, on
the other hand, places an
emphasis on restricting the
consumption of highly
manufactured foods that are
loaded with preservatives and
pesticides.

The Feingold Diet is, in general,
a novel strategy for dealing with
behavioral problems in kids with
ADHD and other conditions.
Limiting the intake of

manufactured foods can be a good first move for anyone seeking to better their general health and wellness, even though more study is required to fully grasp the diet's efficacy.

CHAPTER THREE:
Feingold Diet Breakfast Recipes

Here are 30 breakfast recipes that are suitable for the Feingold Diet:

Day 1:

Scrambled Eggs with Spinach
Ingredients:
2 eggs
1 handful of spinach leaves
1 tablespoon butter or ghee
Salt and pepper to taste
Instructions:
Beat the eggs in a bowl and season with salt and pepper.

Melt the butter or ghee in a pan over medium heat.
Add the spinach and cook until wilted.
Pour in the beaten eggs and scramble until cooked to your liking.
Serve hot.

Day 2:
Almond Butter and Banana Smoothie
Ingredients:
1 banana
1 tablespoon almond butter
1/2 cup unsweetened almond milk
1/2 teaspoon vanilla extract
1/2 teaspoon cinnamon
Instructions:
Blend all ingredients in a blender until smooth.
Serve cold.

Day 3:

Greek Yogurt Parfait
Ingredients:
1/2 cup plain Greek yogurt
1/4 cup granola
1/4 cup fresh berries
Instructions:
Layer the yogurt, granola, and berries in a bowl or jar.
Serve cold

.

Day 4:

Sweet Potato Hash with Eggs
Ingredients:
1 sweet potato, diced
1/2 onion, diced
2 eggs
1 tablespoon coconut oil
Salt and pepper to taste
Instructions:
Heat the coconut oil in a pan over medium heat.

Add the sweet potato and onion
and cook until tender.
Crack the eggs into the pan
and cook to your liking.
Season with salt and pepper.
Serve hot.

Day 5:

Paleo Breakfast Casserole
Ingredients:
8 eggs
1 pound ground breakfast
sausage
1 bell pepper, diced
1/2 onion, diced
1/2 cup coconut milk
Salt and pepper to taste
Instructions:
Preheat the oven to 350°F.
Brown the sausage in a pan
over medium heat.
Add the bell pepper and onion
and cook until tender.

Beat the eggs in a bowl and add the coconut milk, salt, and pepper.
Grease a baking dish and add the sausage mixture to the bottom.
Pour the egg mixture over the sausage mixture.
Bake for 30 minutes or until set.
Serve hot.

Day 6:

Avocado Toast with Poached Eggs
Ingredients:
2 slices of bread, toasted
1 avocado, mashed
2 eggs, poached
Salt and pepper to taste
Instructions:
Spread the mashed avocado on the toasted bread.

Top each slice with a poached egg.
Season with salt and pepper.
Serve hot.

Day 7:

Blueberry Muffins
Ingredients:
1 cup almond flour
1/4 cup coconut flour
1/4 cup honey
3 eggs
1/4 cup coconut oil
1/2 teaspoon baking soda
1/2 teaspoon baking powder
1/2 teaspoon vanilla extract
1/2 cup fresh blueberries
Instructions:
Preheat the oven to 350°F.
Mix all ingredients in a bowl until well combined.

Grease a muffin tin and divide the batter evenly among the cups.
Bake for 20-25 minutes or until a toothpick inserted in the center comes out clean.
Serve warm.

Day 8:
Breakfast Burrito Bowl
Ingredients:
1/2 cup cooked quinoa
1/2 cup black beans, drained and rinsed
1/2 avocado, diced
1/4 cup salsa
2 eggs, scrambled
Salt and pepper to taste
Instructions:
In a bowl, combine the quinoa and black beans.

Add the scrambled eggs, diced avocado, and salsa on top.
Season with salt and pepper.
Serve hot.

Day 9:
Cottage Cheese Pancakes
Ingredients:
1 cup cottage cheese
1/2 cup oat flour
2 eggs
1/2 teaspoon vanilla extract
1/4 teaspoon cinnamon
1/4 teaspoon baking powder
Butter or ghee for cooking
Instructions:
Mix all ingredients in a bowl until well combined.
Heat a nonstick pan over medium heat and melt butter or ghee.

Spoon the pancake batter onto the pan and cook until bubbles form on the surface.
Flip and cook the other side until golden brown.
Repeat with the remaining batter.
Serve warm.

Day 10:

Paleo Breakfast Sausage Patties
Ingredients:
1 pound ground breakfast sausage
1/2 teaspoon dried sage
1/2 teaspoon dried thyme
1/2 teaspoon garlic powder
1/4 teaspoon salt
1/4 teaspoon black pepper
Instructions:

In a bowl, mix all ingredients until well combined.

Form into patties.
Heat a nonstick pan over medium heat and cook the patties until browned on both sides and cooked through.
Serve hot.

Day 11:
Chia Seed Pudding
Ingredients:
1/4 cup chia seeds
1 cup unsweetened almond milk
1 tablespoon honey
1/2 teaspoon vanilla extract
Fresh berries for topping
Instructions:
Mix the chia seeds, almond milk, honey, and vanilla extract in a bowl until well combined.
Refrigerate for at least 2 hours or overnight.
Top with fresh berries before serving.

Day 12:

Zucchini Frittata
Ingredients:
1 small zucchini, sliced
1/2 onion, sliced
2 eggs
1/4 cup almond milk
1 tablespoon butter or ghee
Salt and pepper to taste
Instructions:
Preheat the oven to 350°F.
Melt the butter or ghee in a nonstick oven-safe pan over medium heat.
Add the zucchini and onion and cook until tender.
Beat the eggs in a bowl and add the almond milk, salt, and pepper.
Pour the egg mixture over the vegetables in the pan.

Bake for 10-15 minutes or until set.
Serve hot.

Day 13:

Breakfast Salad
Ingredients:
2 cups mixed greens
1/2 avocado, diced
1/4 cup chopped nuts
2 hard-boiled eggs, sliced
1/4 cup diced tomatoes
Olive oil and balsamic vinegar for dressing
Instructions:
In a bowl, combine the mixed greens, avocado, nuts, eggs, and tomatoes.
Drizzle with olive oil and balsamic vinegar.
Serve cold.

Day 14:

Sweet Potato and Bacon Hash
Ingredients:

Ingredients:
1 sweet potato, diced
4 slices of bacon, chopped
1/2 onion, diced
1 tablespoon butter or ghee
Salt and pepper to taste
Instructions:
Heat a nonstick pan over medium heat and melt the butter or ghee.
Add the sweet potato and cook until tender.
Add the bacon and onion and cook until the bacon is crispy and the onion is soft.
Season with salt and pepper.
Serve hot.

Day 15:

Paleo Granola
Ingredients:
1/2 cup chopped nuts (almonds, pecans, walnuts)
1/2 cup unsweetened coconut flakes
1/2 cup pumpkin seeds
1/2 cup sunflower seeds
1/4 cup coconut oil, melted
1/4 cup honey
1/2 teaspoon cinnamon
Pinch of salt
Instructions:
Preheat the oven to 300°F.
Mix all ingredients in a bowl until well combined.
Spread the mixture on a baking sheet lined with parchment paper.
Bake for 20-25 minutes or until golden brown, stirring halfway through.

Let cool completely before serving.

Day 16:

Egg and Veggie Muffins
Ingredients:
6 eggs
1/4 cup almond milk
1/2 cup chopped vegetables (bell peppers, mushrooms, spinach)
Salt and pepper to taste
Instructions:
Preheat the oven to 350°F.
Grease a muffin tin with cooking spray.
In a bowl, beat the eggs and almond milk until well combined.
Stir in the chopped vegetables and season with salt and pepper.

Pour the mixture into the muffin tin, filling each cup about 2/3 full.
Bake for 20-25 minutes or until set.
Serve hot or cold.

Day 17:

Coconut Flour Pancakes
Ingredients:
1/4 cup coconut flour
2 eggs
1/4 cup unsweetened almond milk
1/4 teaspoon baking powder
Pinch of salt
Butter or ghee for cooking
Instructions:
Mix all ingredients in a bowl until well combined.
Heat a nonstick pan over medium heat and melt butter or ghee.

Spoon the pancake batter onto the pan and cook until bubbles form on the surface.
Flip and cook the other side until golden brown.
Repeat with the remaining batter.
Serve warm.

Day 18:

Greek Yogurt Parfait
Ingredients:
1 cup Greek yogurt
1/4 cup chopped nuts
1/4 cup fresh berries
1 tablespoon honey
Instructions:
In a bowl, mix the Greek yogurt and honey until well combined.
Layer the yogurt, nuts, and berries in a glass.
Serve cold.

Day 19:

Paleo Breakfast Burrito
Ingredients:
2 large collard green leaves
2 eggs, scrambled
1/4 avocado, diced
1/4 cup salsa
Salt and pepper to taste
Instructions:
Blanch the collard green leaves in boiling water for 1-2 minutes.
Lay the leaves flat on a plate and add the scrambled eggs, diced avocado, and salsa.
Season with salt and pepper.
Roll up the leaves to make a burrito.
Serve hot.

Day 20:

Almond Butter and Banana Smoothie

Ingredients:
tablespoons almond butter
1 cup unsweetened almond milk
1/4 teaspoon cinnamon
Ice cubes (optional)
Instructions:
In a blender, combine the banana, almond butter, almond milk, and cinnamon.
Blend until smooth.
Add ice cubes if desired and blend again.
Serve cold.

Day 21:

Coconut Milk Chia Pudding
Ingredients:
1/4 cup chia seeds
1 cup coconut milk
1/2 teaspoon vanilla extract
1 tablespoon honey
Fresh berries for topping
Instructions:

In a bowl, whisk together the chia seeds, coconut milk, vanilla extract, and honey.
Let the mixture sit for 10-15 minutes until the chia seeds absorb the liquid and the mixture thickens.
Stir the mixture and pour into serving dishes.
Top with fresh berries.
Refrigerate for at least 2 hours before serving.

Day 22:

Spinach and Mushroom Omelette
Ingredients:
2 eggs
1/4 cup unsweetened almond milk
1/2 cup chopped spinach
1/2 cup sliced mushrooms

Salt and pepper to taste
Butter or ghee for cooking
Instructions:
In a bowl, beat the eggs and almond milk until well combined.
Heat a nonstick pan over medium heat and melt butter or ghee.
Add the spinach and mushrooms and cook until tender.
Pour the egg mixture into the pan and cook until set.
Season with salt and pepper.
Fold the omelette in half and serve hot.

Day 23:

Paleo Banana Bread
Ingredients:
2 ripe bananas, mashed
2 eggs

1/4 cup coconut oil, melted
1/2 cup almond flour
1/2 cup coconut flour
1/4 cup honey
1 teaspoon baking powder
1/2 teaspoon baking soda
1/2 teaspoon cinnamon
Pinch of salt

Instructions:

Preheat the oven to 350°F.

In a bowl, mix the mashed bananas, eggs, coconut oil, and honey until well combined.

In a separate bowl, whisk together the almond flour, coconut flour, baking powder, baking soda, cinnamon, and salt.

Add the dry ingredients to the wet ingredients and mix until well combined.

Pour the batter into a greased loaf pan.

Bake for 40-45 minutes or until a toothpick inserted into the center comes out clean.
Let cool before slicing and serving.

Day 24:

Smoked Salmon and Avocado Toast
Ingredients:
2 slices of gluten-free bread
1/2 avocado, mashed
2 ounces smoked salmon
1 tablespoon chopped fresh dill
Salt and pepper to taste
Instructions:
Toast the bread.
Spread the mashed avocado on each slice of toast.
Top with smoked salmon and chopped dill.
Season with salt and pepper.
Serve immediately.

Day 25:

Paleo Breakfast Bowl
Ingredients:
2 cups chopped sweet potato
4 slices of bacon, chopped
1/2 onion, diced
1/2 avocado, diced
2 eggs
Salt and pepper to taste
Instructions:
Preheat the oven to 400°F.
Spread the sweet potato on a baking sheet and roast for 20-25 minutes or until tender.
In a nonstick pan, cook the bacon and onion until crispy.
In a separate pan, fry the eggs to your desired level of doneness.

In a bowl, combine the roasted sweet potato, bacon, and onion. Top with diced avocado and the fried eggs.

Season with salt and pepper.
Serve hot.

Day 26:

Blueberry Oatmeal Bake
Ingredients:
2 cups rolled oats
1/2 teaspoon baking powder
1/4 teaspoon salt
1/4 cup honey
1/4 cup unsweetened applesauce
1 egg
1 cup almond milk
1 teaspoon vanilla extract
1 cup fresh or frozen blueberries
Instructions:
Preheat the oven to 375°F.
Grease a baking dish with butter or coconut oil.
In a bowl, mix together the oats, baking powder, and salt.

In another bowl, whisk together the honey, applesauce, egg, almond milk, and vanilla extract. Add the wet ingredients to the dry ingredients and mix until well combined.
Fold in the blueberries.
Pour the mixture into the greased baking dish.
Bake for 30-35 minutes or until golden brown.
Let cool before slicing and serving.

Day 27:

Almond Flour Waffles
Ingredients:
2 cups almond flour
1/2 teaspoon baking powder
1/4 teaspoon salt
4 eggs
1/4 cup unsweetened almond milk

1/4 cup melted coconut oil

1 teaspoon vanilla extract

Instructions:

Preheat the waffle iron.

In a bowl, mix together the almond flour, baking powder, and salt.

In another bowl, whisk together the eggs, almond milk, coconut oil, and vanilla extract.

Add the wet ingredients to the dry ingredients and mix until well combined.

Pour the batter into the preheated waffle iron and cook according to the manufacturer's instructions.

Serve hot with your favorite toppings.

Day 28:

Green Smoothie Bowl

Ingredients:

1 cup unsweetened almond milk
1 frozen banana
1 cup frozen spinach
1/4 avocado
1/4 teaspoon vanilla extract
Toppings of your choice (fresh berries, granola, nuts, etc.)
Instructions:
In a blender, combine the almond milk, frozen banana, frozen spinach, avocado, and vanilla extract.
Blend until smooth.
Pour the mixture into a bowl.
Top with your favorite toppings.
Serve cold.

Day 29:

Sweet Potato Hash with Eggs
Ingredients:
2 cups grated sweet potato
1/2 onion, diced

2 cloves garlic, minced
2 tablespoons ghee or butter
4 eggs
Salt and pepper to taste

Instructions:

In a nonstick pan, melt the ghee or butter over medium heat.

Add the grated sweet potato, onion, and garlic and cook until tender.

In a separate pan, fry the eggs to your desired level of doneness.

Season the sweet potato hash with salt and pepper.

Serve hot with the fried eggs on top.

Day 30:

Paleo Breakfast Tacos
Ingredients:

4 small corn tortillas (check for gluten-free)
4 eggs
1/2 avocado, diced
1/4 cup salsa
Salt and pepper to taste
Fresh cilantro for topping.

CHAPTER FOUR:
Feingold Diet Lunch Recipe

This is a 30 day Feingold Diet Lunch recipe.

Follow this recipe daily for maximum result and remember to keep records each day.

You may need to modify it to suit your individual needs and preferences.

Day 1: Turkey and avocado wrap – sliced turkey, avocado, lettuce, and tomato in a whole wheat wrap

Day 2: Chicken and vegetable stir-fry – chicken breast, broccoli, bell peppers, and carrots stir-fried in sesame oil

Day 3: Veggie burger with sweet potato fries – black bean veggie burger with sweet potato fries and a side of sliced cucumber

Day 4: Tuna salad – canned tuna mixed with avocado, celery, and onion, served on a bed of lettuce

Day 5: Baked sweet potato with chili – baked sweet potato topped with turkey chili and a dollop of Greek yogurt

Day 6: Roast beef and Swiss cheese sandwich – roast beef, Swiss cheese, lettuce, and tomato on a whole wheat bun

Day 7: Quinoa salad – quinoa, cucumber, red onion, cherry tomatoes, and feta cheese with a lemon vinaigrette dressing

Day 8: Chicken and vegetable soup – chicken broth with shredded chicken, diced vegetables, and whole grain noodles

Day 9: Spinach and feta omelette – spinach and feta cheese omelette with a side of fresh fruit

Day 10: Grilled chicken Caesar salad – grilled chicken breast, romaine lettuce, croutons, and Caesar dressing

Day 11: Vegetable frittata – egg frittata with mushrooms, spinach, and bell peppers

Day 12: Mediterranean wrap – hummus, roasted red peppers,

feta cheese, and spinach in a whole wheat wrap

Day 13: Turkey chili – ground turkey, beans, diced tomatoes, and chili powder served with a side of cornbread

Day 14: Chicken and vegetable kebabs – chicken breast and mixed vegetables grilled on skewers and served with tzatziki sauce

Day 15: Broiled salmon and asparagus – broiled salmon fillet with roasted asparagus

Day 16: Turkey and Swiss cheese panini – turkey breast and Swiss cheese on whole wheat bread, grilled with a panini press

Day 17: Quinoa and black bean salad – quinoa, black beans, corn, and red pepper with a lime vinaigrette dressing

Day 18: Roast beef and cheddar sandwich – roast beef, cheddar cheese, lettuce, and tomato on whole wheat bread

Day 19: Chicken and vegetable curry – chicken breast, mixed vegetables, and curry sauce over brown rice

Day 20: Lentil soup – lentil soup with diced vegetables and whole grain crackers

Day 21: Roasted vegetable salad – mixed roasted vegetables, goat cheese, and balsamic vinaigrette dressing

Day 22: Turkey and cranberry sandwich – turkey breast, cranberry sauce, lettuce, and whole wheat bread

Day 23: Grilled chicken and mixed vegetable salad – grilled chicken breast, mixed vegetables, and feta cheese with a balsamic vinaigrette dressing

Day 24: Chickpea salad – chickpeas, diced vegetables, and feta cheese with a lemon vinaigrette dressing

Day 25: Greek yogurt and fruit parfait – Greek yogurt, mixed berries, and granola

Day 26: Turkey and cheddar wrap – turkey breast, cheddar

cheese, lettuce, and tomato in a whole wheat wrap

Day 27: Chicken and broccoli casserole – chicken breast and broccoli baked in a cream sauce

Day 28: Mixed green salad – mixed greens, cherry tomatoes, cucumbers, and shredded carrots with a honey mustard dressing

Day 29: Roast beef and horseradish sandwich – roast beef, horseradish sauce, lettuce.

CHAPTER FIVE: Feingold Diet Recipe For Dinner

This is a 30 day Feingold Diet Dinner recipe.
Follow this recipe daily for maximum result and remember to keep records each day.
You may need to modify it to suit your individual needs and preferences.

Day 1:
Herb Crusted Baked Chicken with Steamed Broccoli and Brown Rice

Day 2:
Vegetarian Chili with Whole Grain Cornbread

Day 3:

Beef Stir-Fry with Carrots and
Snow Peas served over Quinoa

Day 4:
Salmon with Lemon and Dill,
Roasted Asparagus, and Sweet
Potato Mash

Day 5:
Turkey Meatballs with Zucchini
Noodles and Tomato Sauce

Day 6:
Stuffed Peppers with Brown Rice,
Ground Beef, and Tomato Sauce

Day 7:
Lentil Soup with Whole Wheat
Bread

Day 8:
Roasted Chicken with Brussel
Sprouts and Quinoa

Day 9:
Black Bean Tacos with Guacamole and Whole Wheat Tortillas

Day 10:
Grilled Steak with Roasted Carrots and Mashed Sweet Potatoes

Day 11:
Sautéed Shrimp with Brown Rice and Steamed Broccoli

Day 12:
Chicken Fajitas with Whole Wheat Tortillas

Day 13:
Vegetarian Stuffed Portobello Mushrooms with Salad

Day 14:

Spaghetti Squash with Turkey
Bolognese

Day 15:
Baked Fish with Lemon and
Garlic, served with Roasted
Cauliflower and Brown Rice

Day 16:
Beef and Vegetable Skewers
with Quinoa

Day 17:
Chickpea Curry with Brown Rice

Day 18:
Roasted Pork Tenderloin with
Apple and Onion, Sautéed Kale,
and Sweet Potato Mash

Day 19:
Grilled Chicken with Asparagus
and Whole Wheat Couscous

Day 20:
Vegetarian Shepherd's Pie with Sweet Potato Topping

Day 21:
Turkey Chili with Whole Grain Cornbread

Day 22:
Sautéed Shrimp with Brown Rice and Steamed Broccoli

Day 23:
Baked Chicken with Sweet Potato and Carrot Mash

Day 24:
Tofu Stir Fry with Vegetables and Quinoa

Day 25:
Salmon with Lemon and Dill, Roasted Asparagus, and Brown Rice

Day 26:
Beef and Vegetable Soup with Whole Wheat Bread

Day 27:
Vegetarian Chili with Brown Rice

Day 28:
Chicken and Vegetable Skewers with Quinoa

Day 29:
Black Bean and Vegetable Tacos with Guacamole and Whole Wheat Tortillas

Day 30:
Grilled Steak with Roasted Carrots and Mashed Sweet Potatoes.

CHAPTER SIX: Tips for Making Feingold Diet Cooking Easy and Efficient

The Feingold diet is a nutritional strategy created to assist people who have a sensitivity to particular food ingredients, such as synthetic colors, tastes, and preservatives. While adhering to the diet can be difficult, there are some tricks to make preparation quick and effective.

Take the time to prepare your dinners for the week before you begin preparing. By doing this, you'll be able to plan ahead and make sure you have all the necessary components.

Use fresh ingredients: Choose fresh ingredients over manufactured or packed foods to guarantee that your dishes are additive-free. This will help you avoid undesirable chemicals while also enhancing the nutritious worth of your foods.

Invest in high-quality kitchenware to help simplify and speed up the culinary process. Look for equipment that is sturdy, simple to clean, and appropriate for the kinds of dishes you enjoy making.

group cook: If you have a hectic timetable, you might want to think about group preparing your dishes. This entails preparing a lot of food in advance and storing it. You'll save time by doing this and guarantee that you'll always have wholesome food on hand.

Try various herbs and spices: To enhance your food without using fake chemicals, try different herbs and spices. Spices like cumin, coriander, and mustard, as well as fresh plants like basil, rosemary, and thyme, can greatly enhance the taste of your food.

Keep it straightforward: You don't have to prepare complex dishes every day. Simple, healthy dishes can be filling and simple to make. Examples include broiled poultry with baked veggies or a substantial broth.

Keep your kitchen tidy and orderly to make preparing quicker and more effective. This entails marking your components, maintaining a well-stocked larder, and tidying as you go.

By using these suggestions, you can prepare tasty, additive-free dishes on the Feingold diet quickly and easily.

Diet plan checkbox

Write down the meal you take each day under the "meal" column, then write down it's reactions on you under the "remarks" column

Days	Meal	Remarks
1		

2		

3		
4		

5		

6		

7		
8		

9		
10		

11		
12		

13		
14		

15		
16		

17		
18		

19		
20		

21		
22		

23		
24		

25		
26		

27		
28		

29		
30		

105

31

32

33		

Made in United States
Troutdale, OR
01/20/2024

17032867R00066